THE NEW SELF HELP SERIES

VARICOSE VEINS

LEON CHAITOW
N.D., D.O.

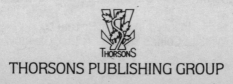

THORSONS PUBLISHING GROUP

First published April 1986

© Thorsons Publishing Group 1986

British Library Cataloguing in Publication Data

Chaitow, Leon
Varicose veins.
1. Varicose veins
I. Title
616.1'43

ISBN 0-7225-1304-6

*Published by Thorsons Publishers Limited,
Wellingborough, Northamptonshire, NN8 2RQ, England*

Printed in Great Britain by
William Collins Sons & Co. Ltd, Glasgow

7 9 11 13 15 14 12 10 8 6

Note to reader

Before following the self-help advice given in this book readers are earnestly urged to give careful consideration to the nature of their particular health problem, and to consult a competent physician if in any doubt. This book should not be regarded as a substitute for professional medical treatment, and whilst every care is taken to ensure the accuracy of the content, the author and the publishers cannot accept legal responsibility for any problem arising out of the experimentation with the methods described.

Contents

1.

The Structure and Function of Veins

The circulation of the blood to, and through, all the tissues of the body is a miracle of engineering. Tens of thousands of miles of blood vessels (estimates put it at 60,000) carry nutrient- and oxygen- rich blood from the heart, and then return it, depleted of these vital elements, and carrying waste products and carbon dioxide. In its journey, blood will be taken, into the kidneys and liver, and eventually the lungs, in order to filter out and eliminate impurities.

The circuit of blood is such that the structures which carry it away from the heart are part of the arterial system (arteries, arterioles) and the vessels which return it towards the heart are part of the venous system (veins, veinules). The physical structure of the arteries and the veins are different in important ways, which we will examine.

All blood vessels, arteries and veins, have an

internal lining which is known as the *tunica intima*. Vessels larger than the very fine sinusoids and capillaries have further layers which surround the lining. These are a middle layer (also known as a coat or tunic) which is made up of muscular-fibrous material, known as the *tunica media*. Outside this lies the layer of connective tissue which blends with the tissues in which the blood vessel lies. This connective tissue layer is called the *tunica adventitia*.

As the heart pumps repeatedly it drives blood to reach all the tissues of the body. The blood is distributed through a series of large tubes, the arteries, which continually subdivide and spread, until the blood is passing through microscopically narrow vessels, through which only a single cell of blood is fine enough to pass. These are the peripheral arterioles known as capillaries or sinusoids, depending on their structure. From these the blood is collected by minute veinules which join together, like the tributaries of a river, to form a system of large tubes called veins, which ultimately return the blood to the heart.

The large vessels leaving the heart have a great deal of elastic tissue in their middle layer (tunica media) which allows for expansion and contraction, as the heart pulsates and pushes the blood through them. The smaller arterial vessels have more smooth muscle than elastic, and help the blood on its way via use of these. The veins have less of a muscular development than the arteries and are seen as reservoirs of unique design, which facilitate the return of blood. The pressure in the veins is much lower than that in the arteries, as a result of the weaker muscular compression on these vessels.

Almost all veins have a system of valves, which serve to prevent blood from flowing backwards. Each valve is formed by a fold, or reduplication, of the inner coat of the vein, which is further strengthened by elastic and connective tissue fibres. The valves are arranged in pairs as a rule (although they are sometimes found in threes, or acting alone) and are half-moon shaped. They allow the free flow of blood towards the heart, but if a backflow should start they become distended, and open out, to stop this unwanted occurrence from taking place. In the veins of the legs, in particular, there are many valves, as the force of gravity has to be overcome in returning blood upwards to the heart.

This return of blood to the heart is governed by several different factors, all of which are important to us in understanding the reasons for the development of varicose veins. A squeezing action is imparted to the veins lying inside muscles, as these contract and relax with use. There is also a degree of pulsating pressure exerted, on some veins, by the contractile force of the arteries which lie alongside them in certain regions. This pressure, and the muscular squeezing, would drive the blood in both directions along the vein, if there were not valves to prevent backflow. As long as the valves are in good working condition there will therefore be a one way flow of blood only.

This question of the competence of the valves is a key to many varicose vein problems. Both arteries and veins are well supplied with nerves, which control the muscular elements of the structure of these vessels. The adequacy of the nerve function, as well as the integrity of the muscles themselves, and the elastic supporting tissues in and around the vessels, are all factors which can influence the efficiency of their ability to function correctly. A further factor which assists markedly in the efficient return of blood to the heart is a pump mechanism which is often overlooked. This is the rhythmic pumping action which respiration produces. As we breathe in and out there is an alternating positive and negative pressure created by the movement of the chest cage and the diaphragm.

The network of veins is divided into different sets of veins. These are the pulmonary veins and the systemic veins. The pulmonary group return freshly oxygenated blood to the heart from the lungs, to where it was carried by arteries. This blood is then pumped out to the body as a whole by the heart. The systemic veins are those that return used blood to the heart. They are in their turn divided into two groups — the superficial and the deep. The deep veins are usually enclosed in the same sheaths of connective tissue which carry major arteries. A pair of veins frequently lie alongside each small artery. The pulsation of the artery can therefore be seen to carry direct impulse to the veins which lie alongside them. The larger arteries usually have only one vein alongside (some have none). Linking the superficial and deep veins are others which go through to perforate the intervening tissues, and these are known as 'perforators'. In many places along the route back towards the heart there occur junctions of veins, which form plexuses, or reservoirs of blood. The superficial veins lie near the surface, unsupported by muscles.

This has implications with regard to varicose veins. Although the entire venous system interconnects, it is the veins of the lower extremity, the leg, that interest us specifically in this study. Its interactions with the mechanisms of circulation in the pelvic structures is the key to much of the varicosity that occurs.

It can be seen that a number of possible factors can influence the condition of the veins and their function. The structural integrity of veins depends, as does all the body, on adequate nutrition. This decides just how well made are the various parts of the machine. The muscular component of the vein, the elastic tissue in it, the connective supporting structures, etc. all depend on adequate nutrition, as does the efficiency of the nervous control of the muscles. Inherited factors can decide on inborn weakness in the overall structure as well. The efficiency of venous return of blood also hinges on such factors as regular muscular contraction, and good respiration, to facilitate the mechanics of circulation.

Who Suffers From Varicose Veins?

One person in five in the UK has, or will have, varicose veins. Most of these will have problems related to the veins of the legs, but some will involve the veins of the rectum, the scrotal region in men and, rarely, the throat (oesphageal veins). The human animal is practically the only one thus affected, and this is part of the price he pays for the upright posture. The involvement of gravity, when we are upright, is a major factor, but should not disguise the fact that varicose veins are rare in societies other than those of the industrialized West. Primitive people seldom have these problems. At particular risk are those who are overweight, constipated, or who have occupations which call for excessive standing. The venous circulation of blood in the lower extremity normally involves blood being drawn from the superficial veins in the lower limb, into the deeper veins, via what are termed the perforating veins. The blood is then pumped from the deep veins upwards, to the heart, by action of the leg muscles (see illustration).

The veins of interest to us are known as the long and the short saphenous veins, as they are the ones most commonly affected. Any factor which hinders free interchange between the superficial and deep veins, or which causes increased pressure in the venous system in the legs, by obstruction, for example, in the pelvis

Fig 1   Venous return in the normal leg

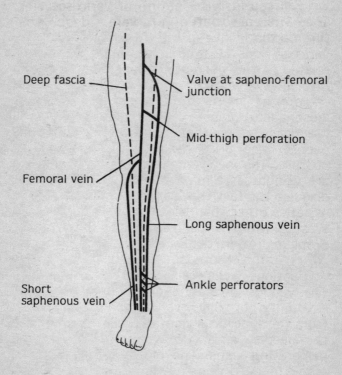

Deep fascia — · · · · · Valve at sapheno-femoral junction

· · · · · Mid-thigh perforation

Femoral vein —

· · · · · Long saphenous vein

· · · · · Ankle perforators

Short saphenous vein —

Normally, blood is drawn from the superficial veins in the lower limb into the deep veins via the perforating veins, and is then pumped up the leg by the action of the leg muscles.

(posture, constipation, pregnancy, etc.), or anything which interferes with the integrity of the valves themselves, can lead to circulatory incompetence. The quality and health of the blood itself is also important in this consideration, as we will see in the next chapter where we will consider the nature of varicose veins, and the associated problem, deep vein thrombosis.

2.

Varicose Veins: What Are They and What Causes Them?

Varicose veins are abnormally lengthened, dilated superficial veins with areas of bunching and sacculation present, which gives them an appearance of tortuous, wormlike structures, elevated from the lower limb, in which they are usually found. They also occur in the lower abdomen, and other forms are found in the rectal regions (haemorrhoids) and the scrotum (varicocele).

The essential observable changes which occur include the following: the vein becomes dilated (swollen or expanded) so that there is an increase in its diameter and circumference. There is an elongation, and a twisting and writhing appearance. There is a loss of elasticity in the vein, and the wall becomes thicker in parts. Those valves which are incompetent may wither (atrophy) and even disappear. The blood within the vein becomes more static and, in some cases, when the valves are in poor condition, there may even be a reverse flow of blood.

The commonest complaint is of an aching heavy pain, and a sense of tiredness in the legs. There may be discoloration or irritation of the skin, overlying the vein. The ankles may become swollen and puffy, especially around the end of the day. In severe cases varicose eczema may develop, as may ulcers, and there is a danger of haemorrhage if ulcers rupture.

In many individuals no symptoms are felt, especially in the early stages of the development of varicose veins. For the majority, however, there is an increased sense of fatigue in the legs, accompanied by cramping, or annoying sensations, and tension or soreness behind the knee or in the calf. The swelling that takes place around the lower leg usually disappears overnight. Women often note an increase in the symptoms described above during their menstrual periods.

The early signs of skin irritation over the veins may be accompanied by intense itching and this may be followed by changes in the pigmentation of the skin, as it takes on a darker or redder appearance. Where the condition is present in anyone who is nervously exhausted, or if there are accompanying emotional problems, the symptoms are usually more marked. There is a danger of an inflammation of the vein itself. This is called phlebitis and we will examine this problem later in this chapter. Women are more prone to varicose veins than men, especially if obese (very overweight) and at the time of pregnancy. Other times when varicocities are likely to become apparent are at puberty and the menopause.

Apart from obesity (when someone is overweight by more than 20 per cent of their normal body weight), the other factor which encourages the condition is an occupation which calls for a great deal of standing, such as that of shop assistant, waitress, hairdresser etc., especially if there is not a great deal of active exercise to compensate for this type of work. Long periods of sitting, such as occurs in typing or office work, also results in stasis of the circulating blood. This can be aggravated by office furniture which causes pressure on the lower limbs, sufficient to reduce circulatory efficiency.

Classically the early symptoms to watch for are a sense of heaviness and fatigue, and changes in the skin colour over the veins. If the sensations described disappear when the legs are raised (they must be at least level with the waist, and preferably higher) then almost certainly varicose veins are developing, even if there are no observable signs of enlarged vein or skin discoloration. Varicose veins of the rectum are called haemorrhoids, and these may or may not produce symptoms. In most respects the treatment for these is similar to that called for in varicocities of the legs. In general the systemic factors which result in varicose veins of the legs, are the same as those which result in haemorrhoids, and the dietary and general advice, regarding hydrotherapy and exercise, will be the same for both conditions, with slight variations which will be mentioned in the appropriate sections.

Phlebitis and DVT

As mentioned above, a condition which can result from varicose veins is phlebitis. In fact, the situation in these conditions is similar to that of the chicken and the egg — which comes first? Many research workers believe that varicose veins do not in fact manifest themselves until there has been the development of what is called deep venous thrombosis (DVT), which it is necessary for us to examine in order to understand the mechanics of the process of varicocity. Other researchers point to DVT resulting from early signs of varicocity.

A thrombus is a blood clot. This may be the result of a slowing down of the movement of blood (sluggish circulation), or to alterations in the actual consistency of the blood. Should the blood become more viscous (sticky) or the circulation sluggish, the formation of such a clot becomes more likely. DVT can also occur if changes in a blood vessel wall should cause a constriction, or narrowing, which results in the blood passing that point being caused to eddy or swirl. Thus anything which impedes the free flow of blood, or which alters the normal fluidity of the blood, can be a predisposing factor in the production of a clot. The factors which can produce these changes are similar to those which are seen as the causes of varicose veins. The production of a clot in a vein almost always results in inflammation of the vein or phlebitis. The sequence of events is difficult to specify, for it is not possible to say whether the clot precedes the inflammation, or vice versa. Nor would it be of much practical value to do so, since the treatment would not alter as a result. There used to be a tendency to speak of thrombophlebitis, or of phlebothrombosis, (clot and inflammation, or inflammation and clot, relating to a vein) but these terms have largely been superceded by the term deep venous thrombosis (DVT).

Once we realize that stasis (sluggish blood movement) or damage to the vessel's wall, through injury or alterations induced, for example, by torsion of the vessel, or an increased tendency of the blood to coagulate, are the major causes, we can see that the therapy has to vary accordingly. The end result of DVT can be very mild indeed, or serious enough to cause death.

Research into the origin of DVT shows that most of these incidents begin in the veins of the calf muscles. The clots can then move on to the other veins, deeper in the leg. It is sometimes noted that veins in the upper leg can be the origin, especially after severe hip injury. The fact that many minor incidents of DVT occur, with no symptoms at all being obvious at the time, usually makes it difficult to be certain of the originating point of the clot and inflammation. Once this has happened, however, the likelihood of deterioration of the function of the valves in the vein affected makes the chances of varicosity much more likely.

The symptoms which may be present in cases of DVT are local pain, swelling or tenderness. The most reliable signs are of local heat or warmth, accompanied by swelling and tenderness. These symptoms may be confused with muscle strain, inflammation of a muscle, muscle rupture, and cellulitis (an inflammation of the connective tissue). Medical therapy, in cases of identified DVT, depends upon what factors can be shown to be causative. Various forms of drug therapy are used to reduce the inflammation, and to dissolve the clot. In most cases this is accompanied by the application of local warm compresses, a degree of compression via elasticated supports, and bandaging and elevation of the leg during the rest phase of recovery. Usually about five days of rest are called for before the patient is allowed to start walking about again. However, there is a fine balance between beneficial bed-rest and bed-rest which can actually cause more problems than it solves, because too much rest slows circulation dramatically, as muscular movement is absent. It should be understood that DVT is a predisposing factor to varicose veins becoming apparent and, conversely, the early symptoms of varicose veins (heavy, aching legs) should be a warning of the possibility of DVT.

Recent research has helped to define different aspects of the symptom picture in varicose vein conditions, as being related to variations in the damage of dysfunction in the circulatory apparatus. Where there are chronic symptoms in the lower limb, other than obvious varicose veins, such as swelling accompanied by a bluish tinge to the tissues of the lower leg, as well as discomfort and aching on walking, then the likelihood is that there is an obstruction of the deep veins. There may be an increase in the pigmentation around the ankle (reddish-brown) as well as a boggy feeling to the tissues, as they are infiltrated by fluid. Ulceration may also be present.

This represents the usual picture when the small perforating veins, which join the superficial and deep veins, are incompetent. This is usually the result of previous thrombosis, which has affected the valves of these veins.

When there is oedema (swelling) around the ankle, as well as discomfort (and possibly ulceration), then there is usually involvement of both the deep vein and the perforating veins. It is possible for all three types of condition to coexist, together with varicose veins, and these represent the development of what is now called chronic venous insufficiency. DVT is the commonest predisposing factor in this condition.

Once either DVT or varicose veins are a reality, there is a very real risk of ulcer development. Many factors can influence the severity of such a progression of events. Some of these are inborn, and it is well established that there is indeed a family tendency to the condition. Whether the cause of varicose veins is seen to be familial, or as a result of DVT (for whatever reasons), the integrity of the skin, the quality of the blood, the ability of the body to heal the local damage etc., all hinge on a number of factors which self-help methods can influence strongly, and which we will consider in later chapters.

The most important factors to be considered initially include the amount of real active movement we perform and our nutritional status, as well as, of course, the desirability of not being overweight or constipated, which factors can impede circulation through the pelvis.

Before considering, in detail, the many ways in which we can help ourselves to avoid varicose veins, as well as how to assist in improving them if they already exist, we should look at the medical methods used. Some of these are safe, and similar to those advocated for self-help. Others are less desirable.

A summary of the complaints which accompany varicose veins:

- Tired aching legs, worse at the end of the day.

Possibly accompanied by all or any of the following:

- Oedema (swelling) which accompanies about half of all cases;
- Itching — this is more common in men;
- Cramp at night;
- Tender areas along the course of veins — these may have a balloon-like feel, and are termed 'blow outs';
- Areas of altered pigmentation on the legs, usually the lower aspect and more often a reddish-brown colour;
- Ulcerated areas around the ankle region.
- Generalized pain and discomfort on standing;
- Elevating the legs brings relief especially from the symptoms of swelling and discomfort;
- Symptoms worse during menstruation for many women;
- Some apparent varicose veins produce no symptoms, and some individuals have many symptoms, with no veins showing as enlarged.

Note: Ulcers may be the result of other factors and these must be differentiated and identified, which calls for expert advice from a health professional.

3.

Medical Treatment of Varicose Veins

Medical care of varicose veins varies according to their severity and any underlying conditions which may be present. Thus if there are any obvious signs of DVT the treatment would include anticoagulant drugs and others to reduce inflammation. The treatment of veins themselves may include surgery, scleropathy, or what is termed conservative treatment, which includes elastic support stockings.

Stripping

Surgery is only really indicated when varicocities are very severe and extend into the upper leg. If a vein in the thigh has become incompetent through collapse of its valves, then surgery is strongly indicated. The operation involves what is called 'stripping' of the veins, with the perforating veins which link it to the deep veins of the leg being tied off. The long saphenous vein of the thigh, together with its tributaries, is divided at its junction with the femoral vein (see illustration) and is tied off. The lower end of the saphenous vein is also tied off.

If the vein is to be stripped a probe is inserted at the lower end and pushed slowly upwards until it is near the groin. A large attachment is then joined to the lower end of the probe (called an 'acorn' because of its shape) and this is pulled upwards, pulling the vein with it. The bleeding which this procedure causes is controlled by firm bandaging and elevation of the leg. Forty-eight hours of bed rest, and bandaging for three weeks or so, is all that is required for normal recovery.

By removing the vein completely the body is forced to produce new channels of circulation for the blood of the leg. This collateral circulation is developed remarkably quickly, and in many cases there are years of freedom from varicose vein discomfort. It is obvious though that should nothing be done to remedy the factors which caused the problem in the first place, there is likely to be a return of symptoms as other veins break down. Surgery is a last option, and there are long waiting lists for those who require hospital time, as this is not seen as a critical or vital operation in most cases. Unless performed privately this is never done for purely cosmetic purposes (i.e. to improve appearance only).

Scleropathy

Far more common, but again not usually performed for cosmetic reasons only, is the

Fig 2   Venous return in the normal leg

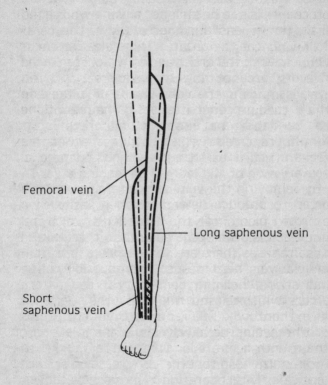

Femoral vein

Long saphenous vein

Short
saphenous vein

practice of scleropathy. This has several advantages as it need not entail the use of hospital facilities.

Scleropathy (from the Greek scleros, meaning 'hard') can be performed quickly, without anaesthetic, in a doctor's consulting room. If the advice given regarding exercise is followed, after this, recovery is usually quick. But this procedure is not suitable for anyone who cannot walk for at least an hour a day in the period following the procedure. This rules out many who have osteoarthritis or who, for other reasons, are not able to walk freely. Anyone who is much overweight is also unsuitable for the procedure, since it calls for the practitioner to be able to identify accurately the incompetent veins which require injection. It is also difficult to obtain a good degree of compression of the leg, via bandaging after the procedure, in legs which contain excessive degree of fat. The method of scleropathy leaves a brown pigmentation on the legs, which may not disappear for some years, and this makes it unsuitable — for cosmetic reasons — for many individuals. There are also other possible contra-indications, including sensitivity to the material which is injected into the veins, the sclerosant.

The method itself requires the identification of the incompetent valves and the injection of these with a material which literally glues the walls of the vein together, to create an artificial blockage. This is done with the leg elevated, and the leg is then bandaged tightly with crêpe material, under which there is a sorbo-rubber material on the sites of the injections. For some weeks after, the patient has to walk a minimum of three miles daily, in order to establish the channels of circulation, which develop to replace the blocked veins.

Support

It is again obvious that if the same factors are present which allowed the development of the varicocities in the first place, then recurrence is likely. This, and the fact that there are many people with varicose veins who are unsuited to the method described (too old, too fat, or unable to walk as described), means that many rely on the standard conservative approach to varicose veins, involving the use of elastic stockings, either below the knee, or extending to incorporate the thigh. These have to be put on prior to standing and left on until bed time. These will not cure the condition, but they are able to relieve the symptoms and reduce deterioration.

Self-help

The above methods (surgery, scleropathy and support) are the range of medical methods available for the treatment of varicose veins. As we will see there are other methods which are of value in many cases, and which include methods aimed at improving the total health of the body, as well as the local status of the tissues of the veins and muscles involved. By improving local and general health, and circulation, through a combination of dietary methods, exercise and hydrotherapy (water treatment) as well as using commonsense methods of avoiding undue strain of the damaged vein, there is a real chance of checking the decline in circulatory competence, which the onset of varicocity indicates.

The avoidance of subsequent inflammatory episodes, and the retention or improvement of venous efficiency, should be the goal of anyone with early stages of varicose veins. Once they are well established the chance of normalizing veins is slight, however, although much can still be done to reduce the danger of ulceration and phlebitis, which exists in such cases.

Self-help means attacking the causes, whereas to a large extent medical treatment is aimed at symptoms. An example of this is the tendency for many medical practitioners to prescribe medication, such as diuretics (to increase the passing of urine) when legs tend to be swollen, and other drugs, based on quinine, for night cramps. The use of diuretics can be extremely harmful, with resulting low blood-pressure in many cases, as well as loss of vital potassium from the body. In the elderly this can also result in incontinence. It does nothing to correct the cause of the swelling, and therefore cannot be seen as effective medicine. Similarly the use of quinine for cramps, whilst sometimes quite useful, is in no way addressing the cause of the problem. The medical approach to varicose veins in the rectum (haemorrhoids) is also directed at the symptoms via surgery, injection of veins, or palliative ointments. The underlying cause, however, which involves the bowels as well as postural factors in most cases, requires attention if recurrence is to be avoided. This will be discussed in subsequent chapters.

4.

Self-help for Early Varicosities

Once valves have become truly incompetent and veins have, as a result, become distended, stretched and tortuous, there is no way in which they can be returned to a normal condition. This makes it critical for the problem to be dealt with adequately at its very earliest signs. If the problem is dealt with when symptoms such as restless legs, swollen ankles, and generally aching and uncomfortable limbs are present, there is every chance of improving insufficiency of the veins, so that true varicosity does not develop.

The Contraceptive Pill
We have discussed some of the causes of varicose veins, and these give strong clues as to the more desirable methods for reversing the process in its early stages. One aspect, not dealt with so far, is the strong tendency which those taking the contraceptive pill display towards the

development of the varicose veins, via the Pill's well-known effect in producing an increased likelihood of deep vein thrombosis. Anyone with circulatory problems of this type should abandon the contraceptive pill as soon as possible.

Two major factors concerning the development of varicose veins are the result of the use of the Pill. Firstly, its use causes the vein walls to dilate, or expand, which slows down the movement of blood through them. Secondly it affects the clotting characteristics of the blood, which increases its stickiness and ability to clump together. This factor occurs more in some women than others. Among the many variables is the fact that women with type O blood groups are less likely to be affected than those with A, B or AB groups (conversely, type O individuals are more likely to have spells of bleeding when they have ulcers than other groups). The life-threatening element of clots developing in some women, as a result of the use of the Pill, should not be forgotten; however the chance of minor thrombophlebotic episodes occurring, with the consequences to the veins as described in the previous chapter, is a far greater likelihood. The first step in preventing deterioration in early varicosities, or circulatory insufficiency, should therefore be to give up the use of the Pill.

Self-help measures
In the same way it is necessary to remove as many factors as possible which might be

adversely influencing the veinous circulation. Thus it is necessary to ensure adequate exercise, and to minimize the effects of excessive standing or sitting, by regularly sitting or lying with the legs elevated. It is vital to remove excess weight and to improve the tone of abdominal musculature, which might have become slack through lack of use or because of postural factors. Use of tight constricting garments should also be stopped, as this too can affect the condition.

It is necessary to ensure that bowel function is regular, and that no straining takes place on defecation. The diet itself should be altered to ensure a wholefood pattern with emphasis on particular nutrients which can help the condition. The breathing pattern should be improved to boost the circulatory efficiency of the body as a whole, and the legs in particular.

Thus with a combination of changes which remove or alter harmful tendencies we have the beginnings of a programme of self-help, for the prevention of the further deterioration of the competence of the veins involved. We also have the chance of actually reversing the tendency and restoring normal function, if only the damage is not too advanced. Other measures which are necessary in the programme include hydrotherapy and the use of herbal substances, which are useful in certain instances.

Exercise

Our first consideration will be that of exercise,

as it relates to the improvement of existing circulatory insufficiency in the veins. In order to achieve a reasonable degree of improvement in circulatory function it is necessary that the exercise involves several aspects of body function: we need to ensure an improvement of general mobility, as well as toning up the body.

The mobilizing effort is achieved by using stretching exercises, based on yoga movements. These are non-violent and cannot be harmful if performed slowly and rhythmically. We must also include breathing exercises, since breathing is of primary importance in restoring circulatory normality. The toning exercises involve any of a number of activities, ranging from walking to swimming, cycling, dancing or skipping. Our emphasis however is on walking, since, unless there are particular reasons why this is not possible, such as arthritic joints, most individuals can walk within the limits of their own current level of fitness.

By regularly using the whole body in a manner which stimulates the muscular pumping action of the veins, there is a profound effect on the total circulatory economy. The exercises suggested therefore incorporate three elements: stretching, toning and breathing, and all three aspects require involvement on a regular basis. Regularity is the most important single factor in the ultimate success, or otherwise, of doing any exercise. This does not mean that they all need to be done every day; however they should be done at least every other day.

Certainly, to gain an effect, whether this be increased elasticity in tissues, with accompanying increased mobility, the alternate day pattern is a minimum. There is no reason why a daily pattern should not be employed, but if this is difficult then the rule should be at least four times each week, with never more than one day in between, for all forms of exercise. If desired the toning exercise (walking, for example) can be done on one day, and the stretching and breathing exercises on the next, and so on. This ensures that the habit of giving twenty to thirty minutes daily to the accomplishment of the improvement is well established. The sequence of performance of the exercises is not strictly essential, although they are given in an order that will ensure that progress is achieved in a particular order, preventing stress on areas that have been neglected in the past.

Stretching Exercises:
Exercise 1
Stand up straight with your feet apart and your hands clasped behind your back. Allow yourself to bend forward from the hips as far as is comfortable. Use no effort but try to allow the weight of the upper body to stretch you forward. Feel the stretch up the back of your legs and especially behind the knees. This exercise is not repeated. You simply hold the position for half a minute, at first breathing slowly and deeply, and allowing the stretch to reach its maximum. As the days go by allow the

time in this position to increase to three minutes. This stretches the hamstrings, helps the muscular supporting structures of the pelvis, and improves abdominal tone if you breath slowly and deeply all the while.

Exercise 2

For this movement you may, at first, need to hold onto a solid object, such as a heavy table, so as not to lose balance. If you can do it unaided, so much the better.

With your feet about 12 to 15 inches (30 to 38cm) apart and standing up straight, slowly go into a squatting position, trying to keep your heels on the floor. If this is not possible then either go just as far as you can into the squat without raising your heels, or wear high heels when doing this exercise. As you squat, stretch your arms forward and lean forward from the waist to maintain balance. If you feel you are toppling backwards you may need to use your hands to balance by holding onto a table or some other heavy object. When you are at the fullest limit of your squat give a few gentle up and down 'jigs', as though you are trying to tuck your tail between your legs. Rise and repeat.

The object of this is to tone the hamstrings but also to act as a general stimulant to circulation and muscle tone in the pelvic area, and to stretch the lower back. When this becomes easy to perform you can vary it by using the more advanced technique of interlocking the fingers behind the neck as you start (head facing straight ahead). At the end of each deep squat rise to your feet slowly, and as you do so stretch the hands (still interlocked) towards the ceiling, pressing the open palms as far upwards as possible. This is further enhanced by breathing in deeply as you stretch upwards. Repeat 3 to 10 times.

Abdominal Toning Exercise:

Lie on the floor with no tight constricting garments. Stretch your arms above your head, so that they are lying on the floor. Press the small of the back against the floor for the duration of the exercise, as this prevents any strain being placed on the low back, which would otherwise tend to arch upwards as the exercises are performed. By pressing the lower back against the floor the abdominal muscles are automatically tightened, which helps to restore tone to these.

Lying in the position described, raise one leg, knee straight, about 15 inches (38cm) from the floor, and slowly start to circle the foot clockwise three or four times, and then anti-clockwise. Lower the leg to the floor slowly. Do the same with the other leg and foot, remembering to press down on the floor with your lower back.

After lowering the second leg slowly, perform the same exercise with both legs raised. When circling this time one leg should go clockwise and the other anticlockwise, before reversing the pattern. Lower and rest.

The breathing pattern during the exercise is important. It should be maintained in a slow rhythmic manner. The breath should not be held during activities of this sort.

After a few weeks of doing this exercise it is desirable to introduce a slight variation, in which, after doing the above movements with the legs at about 15 inches (38cm) distance from the floor, they are again performed, but this time only 3–5 inches (8–13cm) from the floor. This brings other muscles into play and is more difficult than the initial movements.

Both sets of exercise will produce a soreness in the abdominal muscles at first, which is to be expected and should not cause anxiety. The effect of drawing the abdominal muscles into a better position, with increased tone, is the object, and this will be achieved by regularly performing these movements. If a slant board is available there are many other helpful abdominal exercises, but our objective will be achieved by the methods outlined in this chapter, even if no such additional equipment is to hand.

Breathing Exercises:

The diaphragm is a large, dome-shaped muscle, which forms the boundary between the abdominal cavity and the thoracic cavity. On breathing in, the diaphragm should contract and descend, thus producing a partial vacuum in the chest cavity which is filled by the expanding lungs as air rushes into them. During the breathing-out phase, the diaphragm relaxes back, upwards, into its domed position. This encourages the expulsion of 'used' air from the lungs. Breathing in is further augmented by the expansion of the ribs, aided by the muscle groups that control them, just as efficient exhalation is enhanced by the rib cage contracting. Chronic dysfunction and restriction of the diaphragm, and the muscles associated with breathing, may result from a variety of causes including injury, bad posture and emotional stress. Poor breathing patterns are the rule rather than the exception in 'civilized' man.

Breathing is the one vital function over which we can exercise voluntary (i.e. conscious) control. Its intimate connection with our emotions allows us an opportunity to influence the effects of stress and tension for the better, by learning how to introduce a correct, natural, full breathing pattern at will.

The objective in these breathing exercises is to learn how to breathe fully. They can be practised when standing, walking or at rest.

Before learning the exercises, however, one should be aware of the phenomenon of 'over-breathing'. In many people there is a tendency to sigh, catch the breath, gasp, and generally to introduce 'laboured' heavy breathing. Although it may seem harmless to increase the availability of oxygen in this way, it is really this — and the over-exhaling of carbon dioxide — which can produce such symptoms as dizziness, tingling and numbness of the hands and scalp, visual disturbances, etc. It is useful in all breathing exercises to concentrate most on the exhalation phase. If this is adequate, then the quality of the breathing that follows will be greatly improved.

Three-stage Breathing:
Practise this lying down on your back. If the lower back cannot comfortably touch the floor, then either bend the knees, or place a cushion under them.

1. Rest your hands on the upper part of the chest and breathe in slowly, so that this part of the chest rises slightly. Exhale and ensure that all air has been expelled before allowing the in-rush of freshly oxygenated air to expand this part of the chest again. The hands are passive, just resting on the chest and sensing the rhythmic rising and falling of the upper chest cage.

2. Place the hands on the lower ribs, just to each side of the breastbone (sternum), so that the fingertips almost touch on exhalation. As you inhale, feel the ribs expand outwards and away from the body, taking the hands apart from each other. Concentrate on the exhalation being complete, so that the fingertips come, once again, towards each other and the ribs crowd in towards the centre of the body. The next inhalation again produces the sideways expansion of the rib cage as the air fills the lungs. Repeat this 5 to 10 times.

3. Rest your hands on your abdomen at the level of the navel. Inhalation should now commence with the abdomen expanding outwards to allow the downward excursion of the diaphragm and the filling of the lower lobes of the lungs. As this happens, you will feel your hands being pushed upwards (towards the ceiling). Exhalation reverses this, and as the diaphragm returns to its high, domed position, the abdomen flattens and the hands return to their starting position. Repeat this 5 to 10 times.

That completes the three individual stages of breathing. The order is not vital, but after practising these three stages for some days, they should be combined into the complete breathing exercise as outlined below. The speed of these exercises should be slow, they should never be hurried. If 10 cycles of each stage are performed, this would take, at most, 4 minutes, so there must be time to do them even in the busiest day.

Complete Breathing Cycle
This should accompany the performance of the individual stages (above) once you feel satisfied with your ability to do them as described. It can be used on its own as a means of reducing arousal or tension at any time.
Caution: after any deep breathing exercise, rest for a minute or two with the breathing in a natural, uncontrolled pattern, and then rise first to sitting and then to a standing position slowly.

It is not uncommon to feel a little light-headed for a few minutes following the full performance of all the stages of breathing. Simply doing a complete breathing cycle a few times will not produce this effect though.

Lie on the floor as above. Place your hands where they feel most comfortable. Breathe out completely and then start the complete breath by expanding the abdomen slightly (as in stage three), filling the lower lungs with air before allowing the lateral and upward expansion of the lower ribs, to enable those parts of the lungs to fill as well. Finally, complete the inhalation by expanding the upper ribs forward to fill the upper lungs and air passages. This slow filling of the whole chest cavity with its maximum capacity of air, should last a count of between eight and fifteen seconds, depending upon your capacity and control. There should be no straining or tension during the full breathing cycle. If you feel laboured and tensed during the exercise, then shorten the time.

Exhaling reverses the procedure, with the upper passages emptying first, then the lower ribs collapsing gently back to their resting position, and finally the expanded abdomen deflates, and the used air from the lowest reaches of the lungs is expelled. Try to see the process as a bellows emptying. The last air should be expelled with a slight contraction of the abdominal muscles, to take them just beyond their resting position. Pause, with no air in the lungs, for no more than two or three seconds. The refilling of the lungs, following the same slow pattern, is then almost automatic as the air rushes in to fill the vacuum thus created. Inhalation and exhalation should take the same length of time or exhalation should be slightly longer. Repeat this 5 to 10 times, or perform the exercise just once or twice in any appropriate situation.

Tonic exercise for whole body (walking, etc.)
As mentioned above it is essential, if at all possible, to use the whole body in such a way as to stimulate the circulation to its maximum safe level. It is suggested that, before undertaking such exercise, your health advisor be consulted to ensure that no undue strain is being exerted. Jogging is not suggested in this programme, as most individuals requiring assistance for varicose veins are likely to be out of condition, and this requires that the introduction of exercise (of an active type) does not place stress on the heart. Jogging is undesirable for the unfit, whereas walking is safe. Jogging also introduces unusual stresses to the weight-bearing joints of the legs, notably the knees. This is doubly likely in the overweight individual. If cleared by a health professional, skipping, dancing or cycling may be substituted for walking. In such cases it is necessary to increase effort progressively, and this may be achieved by following the methods outlined very clearly in Dr Kenneth Cooper's book, *Aerobics* (Bantam

Books), which is available from good book stores everywhere. This allows anyone, in whatever state of unfitness, to have clear guidelines as to what is required, on a regular basis, to achieve fitness. In general, however, until such a book has been consulted, walking is safe for all.

It is desirable that over a period of about a month, the distance walked is gradually stepped up from an initial one mile distance, to three miles. This should be walked at as brisk a pace as is tolerable. A rule of thumb is that there should be a sense of effort, and that it should not just be a slow amble. Strolling along achieves little. Remember that the veins in the legs require active pumping, and the leg movement is critical. So the brisk transfer of weight from one leg to another, as you step out on the walk, is vital. Good comfortable walking shoes are desirable, and these should be carefully purchased.

The length of time taken for the walk is to some extent dependent on the relative degree of fitness of the individual, but it is to be anticipated that 15 minutes should be taken over a one mile walk. This could be reduced to about 14 minutes when fitness improves.

By doing the stretching exercises at least on alternate days, and including with these the abdominal toning exercise, and the breathing pattern described, a fine start to the programme of self-help for varicose veins will have been made. In addition the walking pattern described gives a complete programme for physical regeneration of the circulatory apparatus, insofar as self-help is concerned.

5.

Nutrition and Varicose Veins: Detoxification and Regeneration

Although nutrition may be seen simply as a description of that which is eaten, it is far more than that. In order to be of use to the body food must be digested, absorbed and transported to the parts of the body where it is needed. This aspect of nutrition, beyond the simple eating of a particular food or diet, is called bio-availability and describes those aspects of a food's progress after it has been eaten. Some foods, and certain patterns of diet, have specific effects on the body as a whole, and on certain individual tissues. Thus we can say that certain patterns will have a detoxifying effect, and that others will accomplish a regeneration of tissues. We will first consider the importance of the process of detoxification in normalizing damaged tissues, such as those involved in varicose veins.

Detoxification
We have learned that the state of the blood

itself is a factor in the development of varicosities. Turgid, sluggish, viscous blood will not be as easily moved as blood which is closer to its desirable fluid state. A diet which is high in complex carbohydrates (which by its nature contains an abundance of fibre) will alter the fat content of blood, and will encourage a more normal constituency. At the same time, such a diet will encourage a more normal bowel function, which is essential if we are to succeed in improving circulatory efficiency in the legs.

The body has a tendency towards health and normality and displays constant effort towards the healing of any aspects which are not functioning normally. This tendency has been called homoeostasis. We recognize that cuts and breaks heal, with no outward influence from our consciousness. We also recognize that there is a natural tendency for most episodes of illness to pass, with or without medication. In the same way we should try to visualize the ever present tendency for the healing and normalizing of tissues which have been abnormal, for whatever reason. The prerequisite of this is that those factors which produced the initial problems should be reversed or stopped. In the case of varicosity we are aware that overweight and constipation are two of the key factors, in many cases. For this reason the pattern of eating which is adopted should simultaneously accomplish a number of ends. It should mitigate against constipation and overweight, and should attempt to reduce the state of the blood which leads to viscosity. Such a diet is described on page 59.

Now it is well established that we are all different in our particular nutrient requirements by virtue of what has been called 'metabolic individuality'. This means that one person may be well and healthy on a diet which would not suit another. This requires that we identify our particular requirements, if we are successfully to reach our goal of providing the right diet for our needs. In this book we have not the space necessary for this exercise in detection, and so will outline a dietary pattern which, whilst adequate for all, may not take all of a person's needs into account. For further information on this topic it is suggested that my book *The New Slimming and Health Workbook* (Thorsons) be consulted. This provides simple sets of questionnaires which enable the identification of individual dietary needs and also specific guidlines to follow thereafter.

The detoxification of the body requires that the following general rules of eating be adopted, and that there are regular periods of restricted eating, or fasting. This latter method provides a dual boost to the body, in that it offers detoxification, as well as the regeneration of tissues which have been functioning at a lower level than is desirable. Our first consideration will be towards fasting, which is the single most powerful healing method available to us.

Fasting

Fasting is the oldest method of healing. It is instinctive in sick animals and probably was in primitive man, too. As well as having psychic and spiritual benefits, if carried out sensibly, fasting can be useful in preventing disease.

Fasting is often confused with starvation but, strictly speaking, it is abstinence for a given time from solid food, but not from liquids. It is the use of liquids that is a controversial area. Some experts say fasting is most effective if it is undertaken on water only, whereas others, including myself, would advocate that fasting should be undertaken using fruit and vegetable juices.

Fasting is useful in most cases of physical illness but there are certain circumstances where it should not be used. Anyone:

— with a peptic ulcer;
— with a history of gout;
— who is pregnant;
— who is diabetic;
— who has heart disease;
— who has kidney disease;
— who has cancer;

should seek professional advice before trying any self-treatment with fasting. This warning does not mean that fasting is unsuitable for these conditions, but it does mean that expert help is required to decide on the type of fast and how long it should be maintained.

There are sometimes some strange things

that might happen to the body during a fast and it is best to understand them before beginning one, so that there is no anxiety when these things happen; they are, after all, frequently signs of rejuvenation.

The sort of signs you can expect to notice are furred tongue, bad breath, dark and often offensive urine, and sometimes the voiding of amazing accretions from the bowels. The degree and intensity of these signs of the body cleansing itself of accumulated toxic waste will vary greatly from person to person, often depending on the underlying health and vitality of the individual, as well as the type of fast being used. Surprisingly, hunger is often not noticed after the first day.

Fasting can be seen as the preparation for spontaneous self-healing by the body. It is not a cure for anything. But it is providing the body with a chance to eliminate toxins which are preventing the body from healing itself. So it is important not to treat the initial signs of fasting, such as a 'sick' headache, with any drugs or potions that will suppress them. The headache will go, and the tongue will again become pink and healthy. All the other symptoms will disappear too.

A short fast may not be long enough for all these things to happen, but by repetition the intensity of elimination experienced with the first fast will lessen, until, in time, fasts may be enjoyed without marked symptoms, which is a sign of increased health. If chronic constipation is a factor then there is a good case for daily enemas, or for those who prefer, a herbal laxative, before and after the fast.

Breaking the fast correctly is also important. After any length of time without solid food there must be a gentle transition back to full diet.

It is also important that during a fast some exercise is taken; staying in bed is seldom called for, but plenty of rest is necessary. So it is unwise to fast while carrying on normal work. It is also unwise to drive during a fast because dizziness may occur. Fresh air and rest are important, as is the avoidance of stress, which explains the popularity of health farms and hydros which can offer a restful environment.

Three-day fasts, done over a weekend, are a good introduction and there is one set out below. But it is necessary to set aside a weekend for the fast during which you drop all major obligations and duties. A three-day detoxification every four to six weeks, over six or twelve months, will produce a dramatic improvement in health in most people. Alternatively you might prefer to fast one day each week. A light meal can be eaten at midday on a Saturday, followed by juice on Saturday evening through to Sunday evening, with the fast being broken Sunday evening or Monday morning. This twenty-four to thirty-six hour fast, every week or fortnight, will be most beneficial to health.

In all cases the aim of a fast is to rest the

body from the constant onslaught of food, and the principles of a fast can also be applied to everyday eating. For instance, break*fast* implies that we have been for a period without food. This is true if the last meal of the day was at 6pm and breakfast is at 7 or 8 am. But if we eat after 9pm then the digestive system will barely have finished coping with the evening meal before the next food starts to arrive. Such a pattern of eating makes people sluggish and lethargic. By eating earlier in the evening, with no snacks later on, you can be livelier in the morning and have a rested digestive system, ready for the next day.

Remember, longer fasts should only be undertaken with the help of a qualified nutritionally-orientated health practitioner.

Preparing for a fast

The day before: a herbal laxative such as psyllium seeds, or a broth made of flax seed (linseed), or castor oil, should be taken after the midday meal, which should itself be light (vegetarian for preference, such as mixed salad or a vegetable soup).

In the evening: have a light fruit meal (pears, apples, grapes), or a vegetable broth (see recipe on page 58).

The next day: on rising drink either chamomile or peppermint tea (unsweetened), or a cup of vegetable broth, or half a cup of spring water with half a cup of carrot juice, beetroot juice; or warm or cold apple juice (diluted with water).

A selection of one of these items, or bottled spring water, should be consumed at intervals, every two to three hours, during the day, making sure that vegetable broth is consumed at least twice during the day (not less than 1 pint/570ml daily) and the total liquid intake is not less than 2½ pints/1.4 litres daily.

If fresh vegetable juice is not obtainable, then Biotta vegetable juice is available at most health food stores, and is suitable for use when fasting, as it contains no preservatives, other than lactic acid, and is guaranteed to be organically grown. Carrot and beetroot are the ideal juices.

Continue this pattern for the two or three days of the fast. Finish the day by eating, on the evening of *the final day*, one of the following 'meals': puréed cooked apple or pear; puréed carrot plus a little puréed vegetable soup; live natural yogurt can be eaten with either of these choices. Chew all food very thoroughly and slowly.

The next morning eat yogurt and grated apple or fresh pear, and have a salad and jacket potato for lunch, continuing thereafter with a normal pattern of eating. Ideally the reformed pattern of eating includes avoiding refined and processed foods, such as white flour and sugar products, and following a wholefood diet.

The advice for ending a fast depends upon the person not being sensitive to any of the foods mentioned. If dairy produce, for example, is in any way suspect then it should play no part in the breaking of the fast. For this reason, anyone with suspected allergies should take advice or be under some degree of supervision during this time.

If it is possible a herbal laxative or castor oil or a warm water enema should be used on the last evening of the fast. If the individual involved is chronically ill, then daily, small, warm-water enemas should be used during the fast. Half a pint (285ml) water at body heat is recommended.

The hygiene of the bowel can be further improved by employing one, or all, of the following during the fast, and for a week or so afterwards:

— daily take a quarter teaspoonful of Vital-Dophilus or half a teaspoonful of Super Dophilus. These highly concentrated acidophilus products will enhance the flora of the bowel, while the Vital-Dophilus is suitable for people who are milk sensitive.

— stir a teaspoonful of fine green clay powder into a small glass of spring water, and allow to settle for an hour. Drink the water, but not the sediment. Do this at least once a day during the fast, and for a week after. The clay has a detoxifying quality and soothes the bowel. Addresses for obtaining these will be given at the end of the book (see page 94).

During the fast
Expect to feel lethargic during the fast, and perhaps a degree colder than usual, so wear an

extra layer of clothing. Rest as much as possible, since the whole object is to allow energy to be employed towards healing, not diffused in unnecessary activity. Take no medication of any sort.

In people of normal weight the fast will result in a number of predictable and beneficial effects, but it won't have the same physiological response in very overweight individuals. For example, growth hormone is released by the pituitary gland as a response to fasting in individuals of normal weight, but less so in overweight ones. Growth hormone has many functions including fat mobilization. Thus, if the fast is undertaken for weight control, it must of necessity be a long fast, and it is vital that this is under strict supervision. A short fast by an overweight person is quite in order, provided their general health is stable (and they do not suffer from diabetes etc.).

Fasting is safe if employed correctly and is one of the swiftest detoxifying and health-promoting methods available. Try it regularly, and you will probably be hooked on it for life — which, if animal studies are any guide will be longer than if you do not fast regularly.

Make your own vegetable broth:
Use organically grown vegetables if possible. If not, scrub well before use. Into 2 quarts (2.2 litres) spring water place four cupfuls of finely chopped beetroots, carrots, thick potato

peelings parsley, courgettes and leaves of beetroot or parsnip. Use no sulphur-rich vegetables such as cabbage or onions, which might produce gas. Simmer for five minutes over a low heat, to allow the breakdown of vegetable fibre and the release of nutrients into the liquid. Cool and strain retaining the liquid and discarding the leftover vegetable content. Don't add salt, as this broth will contain ample natural minerals, providing nutrients without straining the digestive system. Also, it is alkaline and neutralizes any acidity resulting from the fast. Drink at least 1 pint (570ml) of this nutritious broth daily during the fast.

A Reformed Pattern of Eating

The eating pattern which should be followed should take account of the following guidelines, in all cases of varicosity, of whatever region of the body.

• Food should be eaten slowly and chewed thoroughly
• Avoid foods that are very hot or very cold.
• Drinking any liquid with meals interferes with digestion, as does any liquid taken up to an hour after a main meal.
• Simple meals, without sauces, are easier to digest. Combinations of certain foods can produce indigestion, e.g. protein and carbohydrate do not mix well (bread and cheese, or fish and chips).
• Fried and roasted foods are difficult to

digest, and should play only a small part in the diet.

Avoid where possible:
• All white flour products, such as white bread, cakes, pasta, pastry, and biscuits. Replace with wholemeal alternatives.
• All sugar of any colour, and its products, such as sweets, jams, soft drinks, ices, etc. Replace with fruit, dried fruit, sugarless jam, fresh fruit juice, etc.
• Polished (white) rice. Replace with unpolished (brown) rice.
• Any foods containing additives, colouring etc., such as most tinned foods.
• Tea, coffee, chocolate. Replace with herb teas, dandelion or other coffee substitutes.
• Strong condiments (vinegar, pickles, pepper, curry, etc.). Replace with herbs.

Reduce to a minimum the following:
• Alcohol (with the exception of a little wine or real ale).
• Milk, butter, cream and their derivatives. Use only low-fat cheese, in moderation.
• Margarine.
• Salt and salted foods.
• Meat. If animal protein is to be eaten then fish, chicken, eggs, etc. are more desirable than red-meat.

The general pattern of eating should be as follows:
• 50 per cent or more of the diet should be comprised of raw foods such as salad, fruit, seeds, nuts and cereals.

• Breakfast should be a fruit, seed, nut and cereal meal.

• One of the main meals should be a salad-based meal with wholemeal bread or a jacket potato. The other main meal should contain a protein, either animal or vegetarian, and vegetables.

• Desserts should be fruit, fresh or dried. Snacks should be of fruit and seeds (sunflower, etc.).

• Drinks should be between meals, and be either fresh fruit or vegetable juice, or spring water, or a herb tea or coffee substitute, or a yeast-type drink.

• One day each week should be a raw-food day (salad, fruit, seeds and nuts) or a 'fast' day. This should be extended to two days every six weeks or so, as a detoxifying period.

This type of diet, together with regular exercise, adequate rest and relaxation, and structural (mechanical) integrity, is the prerequisite of health.

The pattern suggested will ensure that weight is shed at a steady but not too rapid rate, if this is desirable. It will also help to regulate most cases of constipation. An additional supply of bran (from any health store), of between one and two dessert-spoonfuls daily, will add to this normalizing process. When such a pattern is combined with the exercise pattern already outlined, we have a truly powerful combination in our self-help effort.

Regeneration

Insofar as it is possible to regenerate veins and surrounding tissues that have been affected by the degeneration which precedes varicose veins, the following nutrients should receive our attention, as they have in many cases proved to be of great benefit in this quest.

Vitamin E

The well-respected Canadian research team of Drs Evan and Wilfred Shute have reported that varicose veins improve when vitamin E(d-alpha-tocopherol) is supplemented, at doses of between 400 and 800 IU daily. This, they believe, helps to open the collateral channels of circulation, which relieves the pressure on the malfunctioning veins. As we shall see vitamin E can also be used in direct application to varicose ulcers (see page 92) to good advantage. Be sure that the form of vitamin E used is the natural one. This is easily identified by noting that the label specifies d-alpha tocopherol.

Anyone with breast cancer should avoid high does of vitamin E, as it has been suggested that, in such cases, the condition proliferates faster with vitamin E intake,

Vitamin E is an antioxidant, and helps to prevent damage to tissues which can result, for example, from the oxidation of fats in the body. This has been implicated with degeneration of the arteries, and is a further good reason for ensuring that vitamin E is in good supply. It has a symbiotic relationship with the mineral selenium, and this should be added to the supplement list, in doses of 50mcg daily, taken with vitamin E.

The importance of adequate vitamin E in all circulatory conditions cannot be overemphasized. It is used with benefit in cases as far advanced as gangrene, where amputation is a possibility. This is, of course the very extreme of circulatory inefficiency, and not related to varicose veins directly, but it gives an example of the value of this vitamin.

In the treatment of phlebitis, vitamin E relieves the pain of the condition and prevents clots from forming. Varicose ulcers seldom appear if Vitamin E is used. Although it is stressed that in advanced varicose veins the condition is unlikely to disappear entirely, there is much evidence that with its use, they do not become worse, and there is much less itching and pain, as well as less chance of phlebitis, less swelling and little chance of ulceration. The development of collateral circulation is enhanced by its use, and this takes much of the pressure off the distended veins. There is also the chance of an improvement in the cosmetic appearance of varicose veins with the judicious use of vitamin E. This is a bonus however, and should not be the main aim of the therapy, which is primarily designed to check the decline in the condition, and to prevent complications such as further episodes of phlebitis, ulceration, etc., and to minimize the symptoms of discomfort, pain, itching, swelling. etc.

Rutin and Bioflavonoids

There is a range of substances, which are usually found together with natural vitamin C, with a variety of names, such as rutin, hesperidin, citrus bioflavonoids, flavones and flavonals. These are usually grouped together under the heading of 'vitamin P' by nutritionists, and they play a truly vital role in the health and maintenance of the body. They are, above all, essential for the proper functioning of vitamin C, and when this is utilized as a supplement (see below) it should always be ensured that the label states that bioflavonoids are also present.

Rutosides, such as rutin, which is found in many plants, but in abundance in buckwheat, is noted for its effects on the elasticity of blood vessels. When capillaries are fragile and easily broken, the individual will note a tendency towards easy bruising, and also for a network of tiny web-like blood vessels to be apparent on aspects of the surface of the body. This is called capillary fragility, and buckwheat, containing rutin, is a natural remedy. In the same way the lack of elasticity in the varicose veins of the body can be assisted by the addition of the range of substances which make up this complex (sometimes called vitamin C complex), such as hesperidin and the bioflavonoids. The efficiency of rutin in restless leg syndrome, which is often a precursor of varicose vein development, is recorded in historical times, and is absolutely safe.

Hesperidin has been termed the 'permeability

factor', and has a similar effect to rutin in increasing the elasticity of blood vessels. As a rough guide, about one-fifth of the quantity of vitamin C taken should be in the form of bioflavonoids. It is found in citrus fruit (especially in the pith or white fibrous part), also in apricots, blackberries, cherries, rosehips and buckwheat. It should be ensured that bioflavonoids, rutin and hesperidin are all part of the supplement programme, either combined or individually. Rutin is available as a tea or a tablet.

Vitamin C
The function of vitamin C which most interests us in the context of varicose veins is its ability to maintain and normalize the connective tissue of the body. Collagen fibres, which go to make up much of the supporting structure of the body, including the veins and muscles, are dependent for synthesis on an adequate intake of vitamin C. Vitamin C itself, for adequate function, depends upon suitable levels of the bioflavonoids, as already described.

Many researchers believe that the majority of people in Western society are chronically deficient in vitamin C. Linus Pauling, the double Nobel Laureate, has stressed the importance of an adequate, and regular, intake of this substance, via the diet, and with supplementation if necessary. It is suggested that anyone with tendency to varicose veins takes a minimum of 500mg vitamin C daily, together with 100mg of bioflavonoids.

Vitamin B Complex

It is also essential for there to be an abundance of the vitamin group known as the B complex. These vitamins are necessary for the maintenance of strong blood vessels and for the nerve supply, which governs the tone of the muscular aspect of the nerves.

A 'strong' B complex capsule, or tablet, should be taken daily as part of the programme to assist varicose veins. This means that the major B vitamin such as B_1 (thiamin), B_2 (riboflavin), B_3 (niacin), and B_6 (pyridoxine), should all be present in not less than 25mg strengths. Niacin (B_3) has a specific anti-sludging effect on the blood which assists in reducing vein pressure.

Summary of essential vitamins for varicose veins:

- Vitamin E (d-alpha tocopherol) — 400 to 800 IU (plus 50 to 100mg selenium).
- Vitamin P (bioflavonoids, rutin, hesperidin) 20 per cent of the vitamin C dosage, taken daily (i.e. if one gram of vitamin C is taken, 200mg of bioflavonoids etc., should be taken).
- Vitamin C — 500 to 1000mg daily, with bioflavonoids.
- Vitamin B complex — one strong tablet or capsule.

It is, of course, necessary for all nutrients to be adequately supplied in order for health to be maintained. The specific nutrients mentioned are those which have been shown to have a particularly beneficial effect on varicose veins. The use of these nutrients presupposes that the dietary intake, as a whole, is balanced according to the general requirements outlined in this chapter. It would be foolhardy to ignore the general eating pattern and to hope that taking supplements alone would greatly assist in normalizing problems such as varicose veins.

The dietary pattern discussed previously will aid in reducing any tendency towards constipation, as well as helping towards sensible levels of weight reduction, where this is necessary. The high fibre content of the diet will also help in keeping fat levels of the blood at safe levels. The addition of the nutrients, listed above, will further aid in the recovery of early vein problems, whilst ensuring that in advanced cases the damage progresses as little as possible, at the same time as minimizing the chance of complications, such as ulcers. We will be discussing additional nutrient factors when the problem of varicose ulcers is looked at in the final chapter.

6.

Hydrotherapy and Varicose Veins

The use of simple home therapy, employing water, is a most valuable aid in the treatment of circulatory conditions in general, and varicose veins and haemorrhoids in particular.

The Effects of Hydrotherapy
The main factors that will determine the effects of hydrotherapy on the body are as follows: the site of application; the type of application (immersion, compress, etc); the temperature of the water used; the duration of the application; and the frequency of the application.

There are more nerve endings dealing with the reception of cold stimuli (cold receptors) on the skin surface than those dealing with heat reception. If water of a different temperature to that of the skin surface is applied it will either conduct heat to it or absorb heat from it. Such stimuli have an influence on the sympathetic nervous system and can affect the endocrine (hormonal) system.

Water that is the same temperature as the skin has a marked relaxing and sedative effect on the nervous system. It is axiomatic that the greater the difference in temperature between the application and the skin, the greater will be the potential reaction physiologically. The most far-reaching effect of any hydrotherapeutic measure is that achieved by a short cold application. The immediate constriction of the small blood vessels is followed by dilation and the arrival of fresh blood to warm the area. *Long cold application can be harmful.* A short hot application has a similar primary effect to that of a short cold application. This effect is not as long-lasting as that in the cold reaction. The tissues so treated would tend to become more relaxed and to have less 'tone' than those treated with cold.

Long hot applications are damaging.
There are many variations on the use of hot and cold water, short and long applications that contrast heat and cold, applications that utilize the mechancial force of the water (splashes, jets), applications that involve immersion, and others that involve the use of compresses, packs, etc. The methods we will recommend are those which are simplest to use at home, and which require the minimum of preparation and effort. It must be stressed that anyone with varicose veins, or haemorrhoids, should avoid very hot baths completely, and that all baths

and showers should terminate with the veins affected being lightly chilled by splashing or showering with cold water, for ten to twenty seconds. If there are haemorrhoids present then this can be achieved by use of a hand shower, or by sitting briefly in a basin or bidet.

The following methods may be used as appropriate:

Alternate Hot and Cold Packs

If the veins are swollen but not inflamed, the application of alternate hot and cold packs is advised. This should be done daily, or even twice daily, if the veins respond with reduced swelling and less discomfort. Two basins, and two hand towels, are required. One basin should contain hot, but not boiling, water and the other very cold water, with ice cubes in it. Soak and wring out a towel in the hot water, and place this against the area of a varicosity for one minute. Replace it with a towel which has been soaked and wrung out in cold water. This should stay in position for half a minute. The alternations continue in this manner until four or five hot and cold applications have been made, finishing always with a cold one.

This method 'flushes' the area, and ensures that a degree of fresh blood will have been drawn into the veins of the area, and a dispersal of the blood which which was previously static (more or less) in the area, will have been moved on.

Cold Sprays

A cold spray is another method of ensuring the stimulation of local circulation, together with a toning of the surrounding tissues. A hand-held shower is used to spray the lower leg in a series of sweeps, upwards from the ankle to the knee, so that the area becomes thoroughly chilled, over a period of a minute or so. It may well be that the chilling process will result in a sensation of aching discomfort, as the veins contract and attempt to empty.

Several hours of freedom from discomfort often follows such a treatment, which can be used several times daily if desired. Although veins frequently respond by becoming far less prominent, for some hours after the application, it is unlikely that this response will ever be more than temporary, unless the process of varicosity is in its early stages only.

Local and Waist Compresses

On alternate nights, during the early stages of the treatment programme, and until there is marked improvement in the symptoms and/or appearance of the distended veins, the use of local and waist compresses is suggested.

The method of this combined treatment is as follows: a piece of cotton or linen material, which is long enough to pass once around the waist, and wide enough to cover the area from the lower end of the ribs to the pubic bone, is wrung out in cold water and placed around the waist, and is fixed firmly, but not constrictingly, with one or two safety pins. Over this is placed a slightly wider piece of material, preferably woollen. This should overlap the underlying material, in order to insulate it, and should also be firmly fixed. Over this should be placed the nightclothes, since this is a procedure which is usually employed overnight. Immediately after this a smaller piece of cotton material, similarly wrung out in cold water, is placed around the area of the leg to be treated (over a distended vein) and this too is fixed and covered in a similar manner to the waist compress.

The insulation, if adequate, will ensure that normal body heat will warm the compress, and that this will allow the damp heat to be applied for some hours before the mechanism eases, with the drying out of the materials involved. Should there still be a sensation of coldness after about five minutes, then almost certainly one of the following errors will have been made. The material may have been too wet, because it was inadequately wrung out; it should be applied damp but not dripping. The material may have been insulated or fixed inadequately which allowed the heat build-up from the body to be lost or dispersed, and consequently a chilling rather than a warming effect was achieved. In such a case the whole compress (both local and waist) should be removed and a further attempt made the following night. The local compress on the leg can be kept in place by a woollen stocking or sock if desired. The compresses should be left on overnight or for at least four hours.

The combination of compresses has a remarkably stimulating effect on the circulation through the pelvic and abdominal regions, as well as the leg. The waist compress alone is highly beneficial for haemorrhoids, and can be used on alternate nights for as long as self-help is needed. The cotton material should be well washed before re-use as it absorbs acids from the body.

Sitz Baths

A further method of achieving beneficial stimulation of the circulation through the entire pelvic region, with great benefit to the sluggish circulation of the legs or rectum, is via the use of what is called a sitz bath. This should be performed by using an old fashioned hip-bath. Unfortunately these are seldom available nowadays apart from in antique shops. The following methods are suggested as a compromise, and are applicable to leg varicosities or haemorrhoids.

Run about 6 inches (15cm) of warm water into a normal bath, and place at the foot of the bath a bucket, or other suitable container, in which cold water is placed. This container should be wide enough to allow the feet to be placed in it, whilst sitting in the bath proper.

It is an important part of the procedure to ensure that only the pelvis and waist areas are immersed in the bath, whilst the upper body and legs are clear of the water. The feet are then placed in contrasting water. This position is maintained for two minutes.

Alongside the bath a large container should be placed into which cold water should be run prior to getting into the bath. After two minutes of sitting in the warm water, with the feet in cold water, get out of the bath and sit immediately in the cold water, for no more than one minute. This concludes the complete sitz bath procedure. Ideally some assistance should be available for the speedy transfer from one site to the other and to ensure that towelling is speedily to hand to avoid chilling, as well as undue splashing of the room.

In hydrotherapy establishments the whole procedure is alternated several times, and there is a foot bath of warm water for the period during which the pelvis is immersed in cold water. However the modified method described above will provide a fine stimulus for the venous circulation and will benefit the veins greatly. This procedure can be used on those days that the waist and local compresses are not being used.

Thus on each day there should be the use of the local hot and cold pack, as well as (at a different time of day) the use of a local cold spray. On alternate days the waist and local compress can be used, with the sitz bath procedure on the other days. This is suggested in all cases where veins are permanently distended and causing aching, swelling and itching. If there are lesser symptoms, then a modified approach to these methods must be worked out by the individual.

A variety of herbal and other extracts may be used to advantage in the water thus employed. Seaweed extract, lime blossom or rosemary, are all excellent additions to the water. Sea salt dissolved in the water is also recommended, if available.

Hydrotherapy and Haemorrhoids

Haemorrhoids will benefit by the use of the waist compress, as well as the alternating sitz baths. In addition it is suggested that the area of the rectum should be sprayed with a cold hand-held shower for a fifteen second period, at least once a day, and if possible after each bowel movement. This is suitable for internal haemorrhoids. For external haemorrhoids, especially if they are inflamed, the following method is suggested to assist them back into the rectum.

If the piles are external and greatly inflamed, the *hot soapy sitz bath* is the ideal treatment. Fill a large basin with hot water and add thin shavings of soap, working up a good lather. Immerse the hips completely in this water, trying to work the soapy lather round the pile mass. More hot water should be continually added, and this treatment should be continued for about fifteen minutes. Gradually the irritated sphincter valve at the foot of the rectum will relax and the pile mass can be gently eased into the rectum. This may occur during the first hot sitz bath, but generally when the inflammation is severe two or even three baths will be required before the piles can be reintroduced into the rectum.

Once this is accomplished the part should be bathed with cold water or else the hips immersed in cold water for about thirty seconds. After this, an occasional quick cold sitz bath will ensure that the pile mass does not again protrude. Once external haemorrhoids are no longer inflamed the daily cold spray is suggested for them (as well as after bowel movement).

It can therefore be seen that there are a variety of methods which can, in different ways, assist the healing of the body to restore normality to inflamed and distended tissues. We will now pay attention to a number of factors which require attention in all cases of varicosity.

7.

Summary of Self-help Methods for Varicose Veins

There are many helpful suggestions and tips to be borne in mind in daily life which can minimize the effects of varicose veins when they are present, and which can also lessen the chances of them developing, if they are only in their earliest stage. Not all of these will necessarily apply to everyone but they should be well examined, as despite their relative simplicity they are valuable for most people.

• Constipation should be avoided, and whether or not it is present it is essential that no straining should occur when a bowel movement is taking place. The pressure created in the abdominal and pelvic area, and the consequent backpressure on the veins of the legs, when straining at stool, is enormous and must be avoided. It is essential as a first priority that bowel movements are regular and easy, and this will be much assisted by following the dietary pattern outlined in Chapter 5. The use of dietary fibre is advocated as an extra, if there is any difficulty in passing a motion.

• Excess body weight should be avoided. This requires attention to the dietary pattern as well as regular exercise. It is suggested that the identification of individual metabolic idiosyncrasies are identified, so that the correct pattern of diet is followed for each person. For more information see my book *Your Own Slimming and Health Programme* published by Thorsons. The dietary pattern suggested in Chapter 5 will help to correct weight problems in all people with excess weight, irrespective of metabolic type. The identification of particular needs, however, helps to do this more efficiently, and with more health benefits if these needs are met.

Regular exercise is essential for circulatory efficiency, and the safest of all exercise is walking (see page 45). In order to achieve comprehensive exercise patterns, which will deal with all the requirements of the body in this area, attention should be paid not only to the toning and stimulation of the muscles (via such exercises as aerobics, walking etc.), but also to their elasticity, via stretching types of exercise (yoga, etc.), and also relaxation of the musculature, via relaxation methods.

• It is essential for the efficiency of the circulatory system that the breathing pattern is given due attention. If necessary, treatment from an osteopath or chiropractor is suggested in order to mobilize the physical structures of the respiratory mechanism. This can be valuable if there is a rigidity or immobility of the ribs or spine, which prevents free and easy breathing. Breathing exercises (see page 40) are a useful method of assisting in increasing and maintaining respiratory function, which is vital to circulatory adequacy.

• A wholefood dietary pattern (Chapter 5) is suggested as this will serve a variety of ends. It ensures bowel normality, as well as aiding in maintenance of correct weight levels. Over and above this it helps in the provision of those nutrients which are essential for health, and specifically for the tone and adequacy of the structures relating to the veins.

• If relevant: the contraceptive pill should be stopped in favour of another form of contraception, and avoided it if is not used already. Its adverse effect on the efficiency of the veinous circulation greatly assists a tendency towards varicose veins. Other methods of contraception do not appear to have these adverse effects, which are related to the hormones contained in the Pill.

• Avoid the wearing of tight constrictive clothing, especially if this is around the waist or abdomen, as such clothing will restrict circulation from the legs.

• Women should avoid wearing high heels, as this severely restricts the movement of the lower leg, especially that of the ankle joint. By maintaining a relative stiffness of this joint in walking, high heels minimize the muscular movement which is a vital part of the pumping action on the veins of the lower leg. There is also a tendency, with high heels, to develop a shortening of the muscles of the back of the leg and this can result in increased tension and pressure on the deep veins, which is not helpful to their task.

• The use of elasticated support hose is recommended for anyone in an occupation which entails exessive standing, e.g. waiters, soldiers, hairdressers, dentists, shop-workers, etc. Support hose is also desirable for pregnant women. It should be elasticated or nylon and should extend from the toes to below the knees (including ankle) or, in severe cases, should include the entire thigh as well. It is best to put on the hose before getting out of bed in the morning, as the veins will be at their least distended at this time. If put on later the legs should be elevated and a gentle massaging, or draining of the deep veins undertaken, by gentle stroking from ankle to knee at the back of the calf. The varicosities themselves should *not* be massaged. When the veins are seen to be undistended, the support stocking should be put on. These should not be taken off until night.

The use of support hose is helpful for the overweight, pregnant women, the elderly for whom other forms of treatment are contraindicated, and as a preventive measure for those who stand most of the day. They can give enough support, in mild varicosity, to allow some degree of correction to take place, but in the main they are only palliative and will not cure the condition.

• Local muscular contraction is an aid to the venous circulation to be achieved by movements of the ankles or toes, which causes rhythmical contraction and relaxation of the muscles of the foot, ankle and calf. The more of this that is done the greater the help to the circulation. Periodically during the day it is helpful to lie down for a few minutes, and to perform 'cycling' exercises — legs in the air, hips supported by hands, and a cycling motion performed.

• Avoiding standing wherever this is possible. It is often possible for a person to do the same tasks sitting as standing, and this relieves, to some extent, the pressure of the veins. Much of the preparatory work for cooking can be done sitting; ironing can be done sitting down, etc. If up and about try to keep moving, rather than being static. If this is not possible then remember to pump the muscles of the lower leg as often as possible, by tensing and relaxing those which control the ankle and calf region. Shifting weight from one leg to the other aids circulation when standing for any length of time.

• Whenever possible place the legs in a position where they are at least level with the waist. This should be possible when resting during the day, or in the evening. It is essential that gravity is allowed to assist in venous return and so the legs must not be lower than the level of the waist.

• Raise the foot of the bed on blocks, or books, by about 9 inches (23cm). Surprisingly this is not uncomfortable after the first few nights, and it greatly aids in venous drainage. If this is combined with the wearing of support stockings, or tights, in the morning prior to getting up, the symptoms can be much relieved. Anyone with high blood-pressure, heart problems or breathing difficulties, should take advice before doing this however. The method is particularly useful if ulcers have developed in the lower leg, as long as there are no contraindications.

• If the skin of the lower leg is dry and flaky, then the use of vitamin E oil, applied directly onto the skin every night is a useful measure. This can be obtained from health stores, but otherwise buy vitamin E capsules and use the oil from these. If not obtainable, a variety of creams (unperfumed) are suitable. Those based on the desert plant Aloe Vera are particularly recommended. Washing of the area should be done very gently, and drying by patting, rather than rubbing, is suggested.

• Eat foods containing the bioflavonoids, as described on page 64, concerning nutrients. The pith of oranges is particularly useful. Take supplements as recommended, as these assist in the recovery of normal tone and elasticity.

• Regularly use home hydrotherapy measures, as discussed in Chapter 6.

8.

Advanced Varicose Veins and Venous Ulcers

Ulceration of the leg, when venous circulation breaks down, is not restricted to elderly people. It is estimated that 16 per cent of men and 8 per cent of women who develop this condition do so before the age of 30. As the skin and other tissues age, so does the likelihood of the occurrence of ulcers increase. The sequence of events leading to ulceration is usually as follows.

As we have seen there is a large supply of blood to the leg, via the arteries, in order to feed and service the large muscles and bones of the area. This requires equally large and efficient veins to return the blood to the heart. We have noted that the muscle pumping mechanism is vital to this function. As the ankle flexes, and the foot tends towards an upward pointing position (in walking) there occurs stretching the muscles at the back of the leg and a pumping action on the deep veins which lie inside them, forcing blood upwards. As the foot returns to a neutral position so the muscles relax and the veins refill, ready for the next cycle of pumping. This also drains the tissues of the skin via the superficial veins (which lie outside the muscles). The linking of the superficial veins with the deep veins is the solution to the body's need to ensure adequate circulation. The tendency to a backward flow of blood, when pressure builds up, is overcome by the presence of one-way valves in the veins. Malfunction of these, often due to damage from thrombosis, results in efficiency being lost, with resultant congestion and swelling of the superficial veins. This is the onset of varicosity.

Once the upward flow of blood is slowed down, in this way, there occurs a seepage, or leakage, of fluid into the tissues surrounding the veins. This is most obvious in the skin, as the capillaries enlarge. The consequent seepage from these of fluid results in the deposition in the tissues of a substance called fibrin. The oxygenation of the tissues under the skin is affected, and a 'rubbery' feel is noted in the areas involved. Staining of these tissues by the breakdown of haemoglobin occurs, and the characteristic red-brown tinge is noted. A development of local eczema is common, and this is often followed by the development of the ulceration, after even slight injury to the soggy tissues. The extent of the damage to the veins, and the age and health of the individual, decides the extent and likelihood of the development of this ultimate breakdown in the tissues — the ulcer. This can be a minor irritant or a major disabling condition.

Therapy

Therapy is usually by the use of compression bandaging, which is effective, and this is recommended for anyone with ulceration. At the same time those methods discussed in previous chapters are recommended, and especially the use of oral vitamin E. Compression bandaging involves the application of special pastes to assist healing, overlaid with bandaging which is applied in such a way as to utilize to the maximum the muscular pump mechanisms of the calf (see page 90). Movement and walking is encouraged during the healing phase.

Unfortunately, in many cases, there is a reaction on the part of the local tissues to the paste used, or to the material of the bandaging, and this can present major difficulties as variations constantly have to be found. Infection of the ulcer is a danger, and scrupulous hygiene is required in dealing with them.

It is also essential that the ulcer be given a chance to drain and this, and the specialized nature of the materials used, means that self-help methods cannot always be used in the actual dressing and bandaging of venous ulcers. Professional personnel are best employed, and this means consulting a doctor and having expert bandaging care from an experienced nurse.

Fig 3 Treatment pointers

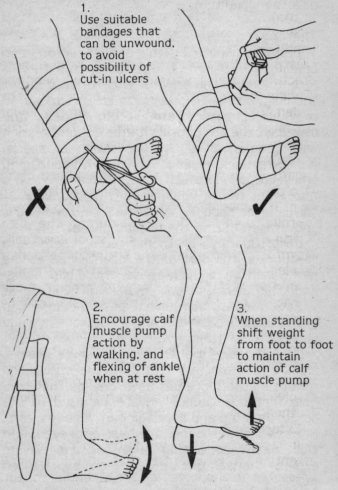

1. Use suitable bandages that can be unwound, to avoid possibility of cut-in ulcers

2. Encourage calf muscle pump action by walking, and flexing of ankle when at rest

3. When standing shift weight from foot to foot to maintain action of calf muscle pump

Active treatment of the leg ulcer involves maximum use of the Calf Muscle Pump — do not encourage the patient to 'put his feet up'.

Self-help for Ulcers

The healing tendency of the body is very active in ulcerations of this type, and it is a sad fact that most complications relating to these conditions take place because of wrong treatment. Prevention is far and away a more practical measure, and this entails following the advice given previously. Above all the oedematous (water-logged) state of the lower leg must be avoided or improved. This is true whether or not ulcers are present.

There is no better self-help method, in this regard, than movement of the ankle to bring into play the pumping mechanism of the deep vein. This should be done before getting up each morning and many times during the day. Putting the feet up on a low stool is actually harmful, as this adds to the static congestion of the leg. It is necessary to have the feet higher than the rest of the body to achieve much gravitational help. Elastic stockings should be worn constantly when out of bed.

The combination of adequate supportive help from stockings (not support tights, but elastic) and the frequent employment of muscular movement, are the best aids to the mechanisms involved, apart of course from the nutritional methods discussed in Chapter 5.

External applications to the ulcerated area will achieve little without such internal attention. It is essential that all injuries and pressures on the lower leg are attended to, and of course avoided, where possible. A slight bump can trigger serious venous ulceration, if the tissues are predisposed. Vitamin E cream or oil can be used directly on an ulcer, and to advantage if all other factors are also being attended to. This can be done twice daily by the simple expedient of puncturing a vitamin E capsule (at least 500 IU of natural d-alpha tocopherol) and squeezing the oil onto the open wound, before covering it again with a dressing.

A dose of 400 to 800 IU of vitamin E should be taken daily. Zinc should be taken in the form of zinc orotate (B_{13} zinc) as this has marked effect on the healing of all wounds, as does vitamin C. Doses suggested are 200mg daily of zinc orotate and 1–2g daily of vitamin C. It is interesting to note that varicose ulcers (as they were called, for they are now known as venous ulcers) were very much more common in the eighteenth century, especially amongst sailors. This was the result of sub-clinical scurvy (vitamin C deficiency).

It has been found in German research that the use of enzymes can greatly assist in the healing of ulceration of this type, and this is a promising future prospect, which is in the early stages of research. Self-help for ulceration involves the assiduous application of all of the methods outlined in this book, as well as the use, if possible, of bandaging in order to compress the venous circulation in the lower leg.

Venous ulcers are a serious possible consequence of varicosity. This unfortunately is a recurrent problem in many individuals who, after months of rest to assist healing, find that they have a new ulceration. This is to be expected if little has been done to overcome the underlying causes of the condition. This is why it is necessary to stress again that all the factors which can be applied from the earlier chapters of this book are applicable to ulceration, which represents the natural progression of the breakdown of tissues affected by varicose veins. It can be said that varicosity represents the ultimate collapse of the veins, in response to the circulatory insufficiency of the leg, and that ulceration represents the ultimate collapse of the skin, in response to the same factor. In this sense both the varicose veins and the ulcer are symptoms, resulting from an underlying circulatory problem, which is the target we should aim to correct.

To pay attention just to the ulcer, or just to the varicosity, is to avoid dealing with the cause of the problem and is to court disappointment. Self-help means dealing with all those causes which lie in your control. Of course some, such as inherited tendencies (a strong factor in this condition), can only be dealt with marginally. However, there is still much that can be done via nutrition, breathing and general exercise, as well as via self-treatment, such as hydro-therapy. (Local water applications are not advised on ulcers, but waist compresses and sitz baths may greatly assist the condition.) In dealing with the ulceration the stimulus to healing which fasting can give cannot be over-emphasized. and this should be carried out as per the instructions in Chapter 5.

Overall much can be done to prevent deterioration towards ulceration, if this advice is followed, and recovery can be speeded. It is largely up to you.

Useful Addresses

Addresses for nutrients on page 57 are:-

Vital-Dophilus: Klaire Laboratories,
                    York YO1 4EY

Super Dophilus: G + G Supplies, 175 London
                    Road, East Grinstead, West
                    Sussex, RH19 1YY.

Fine Green Clay: Cantassium Co. 225 Putney
                    Bridge Rd, London SW15.